CUCKOLD CONVERSION KIT - FOR HUSBANDS

Ethically Getting Her From Wife To Cuckoldress

ALLORA SINCLAIR

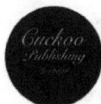

Cuckoo
Publishing

WHAT MUST BE SAID

S o you want your wife to cuckold you but she's not into it? My dear, this is a problem. It's not necessarily a problem that you can't overcome, but it is a problem that may require much time, energy, and commitment, all with the possibility that it fails. This book helps you minimize that chance of failure and maximize the possibilities of living the life that you've always dreamed of.

I do not want to mislead you into thinking there is a secret spell you can cast or a specific thing you can say or do to make your wife want to cuckold you. There just isn't such a thing. However, many women would love the idea of having a cuckold marriage if they could just get past the baggage that society has dumped on their doorstep.

I'm going to make 3 assumptions before we get into the nuts and bolts here.

1. **You've already told your wife of your little "interest" in being a cuckold.**

I f you have this dirty little secret still bouncing around only in your head, it will stay there forever unless you let her in on your secret. Now, I'm not saying you should just blurt out your need to be cuckolded. That would be foolish, you silly boy. But I am saying you need to resign yourself to the fact that at some point, you're gonna need to tell her. The timing for this is very individual and also depends on where you're at as you've picked up this book. We'll come back to this later on.

2. **You understand you CAN NOT MAKE, FORCE, or TRICK your wife into becoming a cuckoldress/hotwife.**

T his is a lifestyle, not an activity. If she doesn't want to do it, it ain't happening. I know this is not what you want to hear but have faith. Many women have a cuckoldress deep within them. This book will help you bring that side of her to the surface to shine and bathe in all the glory of being a goddess.

⚙

3. **You have already done your homework and understand what cuckolding is, what you really are, and how your life and its meaning will be redefined forever should you proceed.**

⚙

This lifestyle is unlike any other fetish. It's not a thing you do once in a while for shits and giggles. It manifests into what you are. A cuckold, devoted, subservient, and loyal to his Goddess.

⚙

I have watched a few of davie's friends struggle like little girls lost on a girl guide field trip, trying to figure out what actions they should take to persuade their wives to consider cuckolding. It's quite funny to hear. If you know in your heart that it has become an essential lifestyle that you must follow, stop playing with yourself and make it happen for real.

As with most amazing things in life, jumping into the lifestyle seldom just happens. It takes work from both parties. Work in understanding each other's needs, wants, and hang-ups. Work in pushing past the original discomfort you both feel, despite the pangs. It takes actual work — as in manual labor for the cuckold. You're going to be one busy girl once your Goddess has made her complete transformation, and understands how you tick. A place where she feels no remorse or guilt in becoming the center of your universe, learning to enjoy humiliating and depriving you as an act of love.

It also takes time and patience. A LOT OF PATIENCE. From both of you. Don't kid yourself. If you're new, you're likely going to feel scared. You'll doubt yourself. Your spouse may move into the lifestyle without issue. And then it will come to the day that she ceremoniously breaks the bonds and cuckolds you. Until that point, you may jump for joy. but then, you'll suffer from your first massive bout of angst. You'll want to retreat and undo all the hard work you both put in to get this far. Who's gotta be patient if this happens? Not you. So don't kid yourself. If you think the patience is lopsided on your end, you would be mistaken. Cuckolding is NOT A THING YOU DO. It's a relationship dynamic and you both need to work at it.

I'm going to state the obvious here, but it's just that important.

Please, please, please, make sure you're ready for this type of relationship dynamic BEFORE you take any outward actions with your wife. This includes disclosing your interest, pampering, self-deprecating, or any other mechanisms to help the odds in your favor, as discussed in this book.

If you're unsure if cuckolding is for you, I recommend reading DNA Of A Cuckold - Husband Edition And Wife Edition before you proceed. With that said, let's dig into the art of seductive persuasion that will ease the transition for your wife.

STEP 1 - THE CONFESSION - DONE THE RIGHT WAY

⚬

I f for some bizarro reason, you're reading this book and you have yet to tell your wife that you want to be cuckolded, I assume you have at least spent a considerable amount of time and energy trying to figure out the what and why you are into cuckolding. If you've skipped that step also, I suspect you are a selfish life partner that will have an unsuccessful transition into cuckolding and likely a failed marriage as well. This is not a journey you take to just get yourself off. The person you love more than anything else is also being asked to take this journey. Stop, drop, and role. Go back to the beginning of your cuckolding research. A shameless plug for my DNA Of A Cuckold series works but feel free to access whatever resource you wish.

With that out of the way, if you have not told your wife about cuckolding, we can follow the first 6 steps of this book without a compromise in ethics or morality. You're not tricking her. You're not forcing her. All I will ask you to do is love and spoil her. This helps prime her mind to being open. Open to a shift in your relationship dynamics. Ultimately, that is the core of cuckolding. What I'm asking you to do is to suspend the sexuality component of cuckolding for a while.

So have you told her yet? If you have not, do it. DO IT NOW! I know it's scary as fuck but it can and has been done millions of times with millions of couples over the years. Leaving this key until later is possible (Step 6 is the last stop for full disclosure before things become unethical without her knowing), but it often can transition unnecessarily rough, unsuccessful, or even worse, relationship jeopardizing.

Do the right thing and tell her. BUT... Tell her the right way.

I've seen so many of our friends fuck this up. The cuck has ten-plus years fantasying about the lifestyle and knows every little detail about the dynamics. To him, this is just the actualization of his dream life. So what does he do? He backs up a small semi-truck and dumps the whole motherload of information on his wife in one shot. She sits there, shocked, scared like she does not know who the hell her husband is, and shuts down or has a meltdown. He retreats and says he was just kidding and the book is closed.

No. No. No. She likely knows nothing about cuckolding. It's even possible she doesn't even know what the word cuckolding means. So, the absolute prime principle I want to impart is patience and always take baby steps.

I'd avoid using the word cuckold (ing/ress) altogether. I hate it. Hotwife I can get behind, but to think of myself as a cuckoldress makes me feel like some kind of spinsterish old hag. The point is to avoid the lingo you're very familiar with (cuck, bull, cage, humiliation, deprivation, etc). It's all about a relationship style that you feel would be ideal to suit both of your needs, in and out of the bedroom.

I would also avoid detailed graphic descriptions of an established cuckold couple until you have two or three conversations on the idea. Telling her you want to jack off while she fucks some random guy in your bed upstairs... probably not a good opening line guy. Yes, you'll get there in dialogues... OVER TIME.

I've found the best transition into cuckolding is to start from the position of saying you want to shift the power and control dynamics in the relationship. Female led relationships dovetail perfectly into cuckolding. Understand, however, you don't want to play that for the next year and a half and then suddenly say you're done just dancing and want to see her have sex with other men. Too late at that point.

A good guideline is to give yourself at least three in-depth conversations dancing around the dynamics shift and then break down the details a little more explicitly. I should note this book is not about telling your wife. It's about coaching her along the journey. The telling is assumed and if you want more advice on the telling, there are many books out there to do that. DNA - wife edition being one of them.

STEP 2 - TIME

⚭

Chances are very good, you have been holding cuckolding close to your heart for several years. Possibly most of your life. Put that in perspective. If you've waited this long, why rush things to get to the finish line once you smell the opportunity.

For some, the introduction to complete immersion of the cuckold lifestyle feels natural and takes little time. This is rarely from the cuckoldress's perspective. I remember when davie and I first explored this lifestyle; I struggled. Not with the appeal or the desire, but with breaking through all the stereotypes and social norms that had been drilled into me since I was a little girl.

Won't this make me a slut? He's going to hate me, and this will destroy our marriage. What will everyone think of me if they ever find out? This kind of thinking is natural even if your DNA makes cuckolding a perfect fit for you.

Please note, I'm not talking about the time required to tell your partner. I'm now referring to the time needed to digest and process the information.

They now know what you're into. What turns you on? What would make you most happy with your relationship and life? It very well may be in total alignment with them as well. But not right away. We, as women, need to psychologically and emotionally catch up.

Be supportive and gentle and resign yourself to the fact that the journey has now been started, nothing else. If you push or pressure them, you're likely to rewind the clock to vanilla forever.

And let's be honest. Part of the fun in cuckolding is the journey. Watching her transition into that selfish, controlling, manipulative, humiliating, sex-starved goddess is... well, I don't think I need to say any more on this, do I gentlemen?

You will get there (hopefully). The takeaway and perhaps the second most important point to helping guide your partner into cuckolding is a deep understanding that it is an enormous deal. If you don't have patience and understanding at the start of the journey as an accepted element that is essential, you're wasting your time. You'll scare her, turn her off the idea altogether, and place your relationship in jeopardy.

You can avoid all of it by understanding you need to not be in any kind of hurry, period. Remember, it takes time for you to fall in love with someone. Instant love is a romantic notion that belongs in fairytales. True deep love demands you know the person. You can't know them without passaging time. We can say the same with bringing your partner into the cuckolding lifestyle. You need to give them time to open their heart and mind to a lifestyle that may be out there from what they're used to, but in reality is much better suited to their needs, your needs, and your shared relationship.

STEP 3 - MORE TIME

A key point that can not be stated enough is that cuckolding is not just about fucking. It's about the dynamic a couple shares. It's about loving each other so much that you both push past the surface-level relationship stuff that most never get past, and jump into the darker side of yourselves.

You both feed each other a side that you would never consider acceptable under normal circumstances. And this accentuates the love you have for that person. This is a massive shift from vanilla.

But remember, the sex component is the final pay-off. It's the reward you give each other. You gave her the gift of having unlimited orgasms. She gave you the gift of denial from those orgasms. It's the endgame. But it's only the end game.

As I've said, cuckolding is a dynamic. Even the word dynamic says it all.

"Characterized by constant change, activity or progress."

English? Dynamic is a journey NOT AN END GAME! Sex is just a small part of the lifestyle. I get so frustrated and angry with the volume of information out there that focuses on the sex only. If that's all your after, cuckolding is a true waste of your time and your spouses'. Check out some hotwife information and be gone, little girl. Stop wasting your time thinking you want to be cuckolded. What you want is to pimp your wife out so you can have a real-life porn theater. Not saying there's anything wrong with that, but it ain't cuckolding my love.

The reiteration of the time element for two consecutive chapters is to drive the point.

Enjoy the changes as they evolve, regardless of the sex that happens. If you've done everything right and it appeals to her, you'll get there.

Sometimes, you both may discover that the sex part is not what you both want and need. You just want an FLR relationship where she's the boss. Sometimes you may discover that you, yourself, don't want to go all the way once you implement disparity in other parts of your relationship.

Most often, as you both shift and change, things get more comfortable and natural for both of you and the sex she has with other men drives a bond so deep, neither of you could ever imagine how you lived any other way.

Regardless of the outcome, moving slowly is not just about the outward actions you do or don't take. It's about the time required for the mind and heart to keep up with those changes. If things are not in sync, it often blows up in your face.

With davie and me, he pushed way too hard at first. It turned me off because of how excited and eager he was to see me suck another man's cock. It made me feel like a prostitute. Fortunately for him, my libido was too big to care much. But I do remember the negative feelings. I just don't want to see other women feeling this way when they don't have to. If you're gentle with your words and expectations, the reality comes a lot quicker than if you push.

STEP 4 - FORCE THE SHIFT

꙳

The title must have you scratching your head, thinking this woman is nuts. She just told me to be patient, go gentle and slow, and don't force it. Now she's saying to force the shift? WTF?

Yes. And no. Yes, it is a little confusing and appears to contradict, but NO, I'm not suggesting you force your partner into this lifestyle, UNDER ALL AND ANY CIRCUMSTANCES.

I am suggesting you force yourself to make changes BEFORE she makes any herself. Not change to your relationship or expectations. I'm talking about changes within and about yourself.

How can you ask or expect your spouse to do things they have been taught from childhood not to do, if you don't do the same... preferably first? You want her to humiliate you, right? You want her to tell you that you're useless in bed and that she wants a real man's cock, right?

You want her to be unapologetically selfish with her life-style choices, right? Don't you think it makes sense you help her by changing yourself first?

The easiest and non-objectionable way to shift power and start setting up the disparity in your relationship is to change the day-to-day expectations and routines. Be open and honest with her, you want to be cuckolded, but that you appreciate this is a big step for her to take.

Clarify that cuckolding is about the dynamics and the power shift, not just the sex. Polish this off by suggesting you establish at least at some level, an FLR (female-led relationship). This enables her to wear the pants and for you to slip on the skirt, metaphorically (or literally, if that's your thing :)

This can be done with ease and requires no effort on her behalf. If you are debating what to have for dinner, she wins. What movie to watch, her choice ALWAYS. If you're in some kind of dispute over anything, step to the side, apologize (even if you're right), and let her have her way. Did I mention, ALWAYS? Empowerment is your friend.

The more compliant you become to her every whim, the easier it becomes for her to not only feel in charge but also to get used to it and enjoy it. Your end game is not as obvious as you may think. Her adaptation to getting her way, though very sweet, is lost with a slip-up on your end.

That is... unless it becomes an expectation. Once she comes to expect being treated like a Goddess in your daily life as a couple, when you slip up (and you will), she will not tolerate the dissension. Over time, it becomes part of who she is and a part of who you are inside your relationship. This is one of the last steps before you step outside of actions that are within your control.

Just like no one has to think about breathing, you just do it naturally. You want to put your cuckoldress in the headspace. If total power and control are only in her hands, it is what it is. Over time, it becomes the norm without thinking.

STEP 5 - SPEND, SPEND, SPEND

T his is when the real fun begins. Not one of my female friends has ever objected to or felt uncomfortable with this. Money. Yours. Spent on her to spoil and pamper herself. I'm not talking about showing up at the door with a dozen red roses or a box of chocolates. Ew, gross. That's the bull's job (lol).

I'm talking about giving her the encouragement, support, and unconditional freedom to go out and spend. Spend on anything and everything that will make her feel hotter, sexier, more attractive. Make-up, hair, clothes, gym membership, tanning salon, breast enlargement (if she wants it) Whatever you got.

Fortunately for me, davie's job provides us both well. I don't work (besides my microscopic contribution to writing these books to help other couples), so he carries the financial weight of our household 99.9% on his own. I am very sensitive to the fact that some of you little cucks are not in the same financial position. The worst thing you could do is get your family in financial crisis to help move your wife along into this dynamic.

If you are limited with funds, don't over-extend yourself in debt. But what you can do is cut back on everything spent on yourself. Channel all the money towards her. All of it. Besides food and bills, she should see every drop of disposable income in her purse.

I'm not promoting the findom lifestyle, to be clear. What I am suggesting is you do whatever is within your financial means to spend, spoil and pamper her. Just take a minute and think this through. What are you going to achieve by doing this? Think long-term, little men. Long term. Not short-term, live out a sexual fantasy and you're done. This, all of it. Every drop of it. It's all about the long game. Cuckolding as I've said is not a quick and easy event. If you think it is, you're in the wrong book. When you look long-term at this spending and spoiling, it has a two-fold effect.

First, it reinforces step 4, only now, it's not just chores and decisions. Now it's the last resource that you have available to you as a man. If your spouse has access, control, and engagement in the spending of the cold hard dollar, you become functionally... like your little pee-pee - useless. I say this tongue in cheek. Clearly, you're not useless. You both provide an emotional, loving connection to each other. But the acceptance that you are her little bitch boy is inevitable and sought after by both of you. Doing these steps just helps her get there a little easier.

The second component of financial disparity is a little more obvious. You want your wife to cuckold you, right? Which fairly sure means you want her to attract the attention of other men? You want her to feel on top of the world at all times, no? New hairdo, expensive high-quality make-up, new sexy shoes, constantly evolving and increasingly daring little sexy outfits. What do you think that's going to do to a woman?

I know for me; it took me a few months to feel the part. But boy, did this help to accelerate the growth in my head. It didn't take me long to embrace this part of cuckolding. Frankly, this would be one of the hardest things to give up if davie ever reconsidered.

STEP 6 - LET'S WATCH THIS TOGETHER

⚥

W e're here. Step 6. This is the turning point. This is where you have zero options. You could follow the previous 5 steps and still leave your spouse in the dark about your cuckolding desires. Until now, all you've done is made her life easier and spoiled her rotten. But here? In step 6? No more.

If you have read this far and have for some flawed reason, held off in talking, now is the time. Going forward, I'm assuming your spouse is aware of cuckolding and has had ample time to digest it. Beware, the time to do that can be months, so I have warned you.

Also, I'm assuming that your spouse is not only aware of your cuckolding desires, but she also has remained open to the possibilities. She may have not given the green light (that's what steps 1-5 help her through) but she is aware and has not given you a hard "no" as her response. IF SHE HAS SAID NO, it's over. You're done. Cuckolding is not in your relationship cards. And that's okay. You can still find other ways to feed your needs that your wife may be more open to. But cuckolding will not happen. Failure to understand and respect that is flagrant spousal abuse (whether it's physical, mental, or emotional). Not cool gentlemen. If you can't let it go, I encourage both of you to talk about it openly in the company of a trained therapist. There are always solutions. Sometimes, we just need the help of a professional.

That all said, now you want to take the reality in your head and help it slide into your spouse's. I'm not talking about the disparity dynamic. Now we are looking at the payoffs in the sexual world. To be officially cuck'd.

Be sure to preview your selections before sharing them with your wife. There is a ton of crappy, fake, and/or badly acted out cuckolding videos. There are, however, several very good porn videos that offer some insight into the scene of experiencing a bull, the role the cuck takes, and the pleasure, power, and control the cuckoldress is given.

Though I'm sure davie has had a lot more experience with this than I have, I'd recommend you try to find the amateur clips only. The film quality is dodgy but there is no acting. It's raw, real fun, and exciting. And that's what you both should experience as well.

Let your wife see how it excites you. Now is not the time to get all shy. Don't be afraid to say you like this or that in a particular scene. Let her know you like being the guy behind the camera filming or pleasing yourself while she gets pounded. If you want to be sissified or humiliated and that comes on the screen, be brave. She can't read your friggen mind. Vocalize that it turns you on.

Also, ask her what her thoughts are. Is she getting

excited? Could she see herself doing some things you're watching together? Watching cuck porn together will instigate both thought and dialogue. This is the intention. You want to talk more openly about the mechanics of cuckolding in the bedroom. This is where you are likely to have the greatest opposition.

Now that she has had time to digest and feel comfortable with most of the other components of the dynamic, the outside world of other men is the last frontier. Using porn should help you leverage the conversation to talk about those uncomfortable areas of your sex life.

To add spice to the mix, consider stimulating her WHILE THE PORN is playing. Ask her to imagine the experiences on the monitor/TV screen while she is experiencing the sexual pleasures in real life. Often, this is enough to bounce you out of discussion straight into the real deal. If not, this step takes things up a level but still maintains zero threat to either of you doing something that can't be undone down the road.

STEP 7 - DID YOU SEE THAT GUY LOOK AT YOU?

S peaking from personal experience, this was the first step that davie and I took that helped me the most. Until this happened, I just couldn't get past it. I mean, don't think for one second I wasn't into the idea of becoming a cuckoldress. As soon as I found out that it was not only a possibility but that davie was into it, it sold me.

What I struggled with the absolute most, though, was hurting the man that I love more than anything else in the world. Sure, I could let him pamper and spoil me. I could even enjoy the videos and I had no problems with my imagination. But going out and fucking another man in front of my husband. Ouch! So, we took it in microscopic doses. This step is no longer thinking or talking or considering. This is the first real-life doing step. Other men. Real men in the real world.

It started with davie bringing my attention to other

men that would look at me in my new little outfits. Yes, I intentionally started dressing to impress, but I still felt guilty acknowledging any man besides davie. But when he mentioned it, it made the guilt feel a little less. Like he knew about it and was ok with it.

This can become a little game between the two of you. See who catches the most men starring, lusting, wanting to have her. As the saying goes, practice makes perfect. Do this with your goddess enough. She not only notices it more herself but also looks for it.

One small step later, you find your wife now looking at other men and making comments of any kind. Yes, first the game becomes you noticing other men looking at her, then she notices and makes comments too. But the "real" real fun is just beginning.

Communicate that you not only like that she notices others looking at her, but that you would love it if she returned the favor. If she sees a guy she "admires", she should let you know. The more guys, the better. This can shift her comfort to look and vocalize interest quicker than you think.

The point in this somewhat innocent exercise is to help her gain confidence with other men besides you looking at her, but also to shift her attention away from you and out to other men. She's not doing anything other than window shopping. But until now, it's all been in your heads. As you both get comfortable vocalizing that other men are looking at her and that she is looking at, her guilt to notice and think beyond what's between your legs is less of a tremendous step. This is not a big step. But it's a step.

Don't kid yourself. This sounds like an over-simplified and straightforward decision. If your woman has an interest in cuckolding but is still scared and reluctant, this step makes things a quantum leap easier down the road. Remember, you want her journey to feel natural, comfortable, unthreatening, and of her own choice. This is an under-valued but essential step that often is overlooked or bypassed, making later shifts into the lifestyle feel clunky, forced, and confusing to both your realities.

STEP 8 - SELF DEPRIVATION

Keeping on the same theme of outward changes, you need to make some changes of your own. Until now, you have shifted your time, energy, and attention to your soon-to- be cuckoldress. You have created a vanilla world of disparity in the household and now she has left vanilla a small amount by feeling confident in telling you she finds this guy or that guy hot, or that she would love to see how he would be in bed.

Now it's your turn to crank the disparity dial up a notch... in the bedroom. Everything in the bedroom you have left unchanged, mostly. Yes, you've looked at cuckold porn together and played with the ideas in your minds. But now you get to play with it further.

Now you make every human effort to give up on sexual gratification FOR YOURSELF. You want her pleasure to be the only thing that matters AS MUCH AS POSSIBLE.

Does this mean you can't get off? No, silly. You have a hand.

But you want her to stop thinking of you to be satisfied, at least, not using your little pee-pee. Your hands, mouth, toys. A girls' gotta have fun. But no more. Consider "sex" as everything but sex. The more you can help her reach orgasm without it being a mutual act, the more she will detach from you as her key sexual partner.

Over time, with continued self-denial, she will begin to feel like she loves you for being so selfless and giving AND the more she will feel like she no longer has a sexual partner that will satisfy her cravings. Can you see what's happening here? This is the foundation of what is about to come for both of your realities.

After a short time of you denying yourself, she is likely to question why? Do you not find her attractive or sexy? DO NOT LIE OR TRY TO DECEIVE. Be open and honest. Tell her you want her to become selfish. Don't be ashamed or afraid to discuss that you have an ulterior motive. That you want her to feel the need to fuck and that you want to feel deprived.

Expect this to be met with confusion and/or objections. She will want to feel wanted. She will want you to want her sexually. Talk about this kind of thing as it comes up (and it will). I felt sure davie was looking to divorce me. Like I was not good enough.

The more I cared and tried to seduce him to have sex, the more he must have manifested thoughts of his grandmother. He seemed to make himself soft. Maybe he was suffering ED or relieved himself just before we were intimate? I don't know, but he just couldn't do the job. What he could do was use his mouth, get me off, and then he'd want to snuggle. Who does that?

Men, you know who! A little sissy cuck like yourself does.

The more you repeat this pattern of your spouse having sexual pleasure, satisfaction and for both of you to feel comfortable with you having nothing, the closer you are setting the stage. The most appropriate word is NORMALIZATION. You want this lack of intercourse to think and feel normal for both of you.

The end game of this step is essential. Your goal is to open the door for your Goddess to think of you as insufficient in fulfilling the male sexuality component of your relationship. Understand, this does not mean that she will stop loving you or stop looking at you as the man who has her back at all times. You just want to become the man she no longer thinks of pleasing her sexual needs.

Again, this may take time for your relationship to shift into this sphere of normality, but that's okay. You are still both very much in the world of doing nothing beyond each other. Nothing done so far can't be undone. Make sure you discuss this with her. Tell her as you leave this step that this is what you are hoping to achieve. That you want to make sure she feels okay with your relationship this way. If she objects, do not move forward. This is pivotal. There is no way in hell she is going to be okay fucking another man in front of you, with you locked in your tiny cage without first being able to have an orgasm, turn around, kiss you good night, and you're solo.

STEP 9 - YOUR NOT MAN ENOUGH

For any woman to enter cuckolding, several things need to be in place. She has to feel safe and secure that you love her NO MATTER WHAT. She has to have a high libido/sex drive (if this is not in place, open a lifetime membership to your favorite porn site, cause you're shit out of luck, honey). Furthermore, she has to have her own self-identity and values in alignment (she is comfortable not sticking to the boring values that the vanilla world has imposed on her since birth). She has to have a sadistic core (also mandatory for any long term success in this lifestyle). And here's the big one... she has to want to fuck other men BECAUSE SHE WANTS TO, NOT BECAUSE YOU WANT HER TO. This step is the last subtle step to get her the rest of the way in her head and heart on board.

So far, if you have followed each step carefully and thoroughly, she will almost be there. But there is still the question of you and how she looks at you. She may have opened her mind to other men and to have a lop-sided relationship with you in almost every area. But you're still the "man". The man. The guy she said, "I do". You can't be that man anymore, cause you DON'T DO. The doing needs to be passed off to a real man.

Getting her to think of you in this light is perhaps the biggest challenge that you will face for yourself. You need to step back from the role of being the man. We both know what you really are. You are not the man, you're the teeny weeny polka dot bikini little cutesy boy that is there to serve and protect his goddess.

Am I wrong, girls?

You know it. I know it. Now we need your wife to feel it, think it and ultimately, to EMBRACE IT.

By paving the way in all the eight previous steps, you may be unaware, but you are building up her ego, confidence, and sexual desire. You've normalized the disparity in both your heads. Given enough time, it just feels right for both of you she is THE GODDESS and you are there to serve... the way it should be. This shift also helps her think in terms of what she actually deserves (not just wants). Once it feels normal, and she wants the dynamic to change so a real man can fuck her hard, you're only a few breaths away.

Let me introduce you to two of your best friends. Sissification and feminization. They will help you, hold you, caress you and lead you to that special, soft secret place in your cuckoldress's heart. It will help her make the final transition over to being the goddess you both know she was born to be, and you were born to serve.

Every chance you get, lose the man. Does something need fixing? Call someone else in to fix it. Need something moved? Struggle. Vocalize your pain. Asked for an opinion? Indecisiveness is your friend here. You want to become the opposite of what a stereotypical man represents.

Take care of your personal grooming more than the average guy. Perhaps go to the nail salon WITH your Goddess. Get a manicure and pedicure together. Not saying you have to have your nails colored (clear is fine), but become besties.

Clothes? Learn to shine. A plain T-shirt and bummy jeans are for real men. You want to wear proper slacks and a nice, stylish shirt that says you've taken time to look good. Same with your hair. Think about getting it colored/bleached?

The point is, you want to be seen by your wife/partner as having little manly attributes. This does not happen overnight, particularly if you've always been the guy to watch the Sunday night football and hang with your bros in the garage fixing cars. Not saying you can't still enjoy those things, but you are re-inventing yourself. You are becoming her little princess. This CAN NOT happen if you're still seen as a real man.

You also need to drop the male bravado. Gentle, kind, non-aggressive, compliant. Not something I think most guys dream of becoming as they grow up. In your case, this is your dream come true. You know this is the real you hiding for so many years. Chances are you've hated being "the man". You want to be soft and gentle, like a little flower, right? Come on, girls, face it. So stop fighting yourself. Let your partner see that side. The girly side that you want to let out.

I'm not saying you are a closet homosexual, transvestite, or whatever. I am saying you are not a REAL

MAN. You are a man that loves, respects, serves. But the real men are out there waiting to fuck us proper. That is not your job - it's theirs. You know it. You want it. So start acting like it.

Don't be afraid of self-deprecation. "I'm useless as a lover." "I catch like a girl." "I think my thighs are getting too fat." Anything you can say to help her transition in her mind is awesome, and she is lucky to have you as her little devout cucky boy.

All real cucks are the same. You love to be humiliated, used, abused, and, frankly, treated like little girls. I don't blame you. I think this is fantastic! But how do you expect your Goddess to treat you this way if you hang on to the man's man facade? Help her. Make it easier for her to transition. If you are more than halfway to being a sissy without her doing anything, it becomes almost natural for her to treat you like one. You deserve to be treated like a sissy if everything about you screams "I'm a delicate flower. Please be gentle with my hair."

You get my point.

The important thing to remember is despite your sissy side, NEVER lose your outward love and protective side in the relationship. Yes, over time you will become feminized, but your Goddess is your partner. It is your duty and responsibility to protect her. She needs to know WITH NO DOUBT if push comes to shove; you have her back and will do whatever it takes to protect her.

You're her puppet, her best friend, but you're also the man she loves and wants to be loved by. Make sure you never ever lose that. Easier said than done. Trust me.

STEP 10 - USE YOUR WORDS SELFISHLESSLY

Yes, I've made a new word in the English language - "Selfishlessly". Now is the ideal time to reopen the pandora's box of cuckoldry in conversation. So far, you've talked. Then you've made some personal changes to revere her and diminish yourself. You've then helped her go outside her comfort zone and see other men as a real possibility, all the while bolstering her self-confidence, expectations, and views on who you are. She is very close to the edge. Closer than you think (believe me, I was that woman once).

She needs to be told that you have loved the journey you have taken. That she has accepted you for who you are. BUT NOW (assuming she has made some ground in her own journey) you also need to reaffirm how much you've loved to see the changes she has made in herself.

If she now feels comfortable talking about other men and how she finds them sexy, tell her you love when she does it. That it excites you. When she dresses up in public, don't be afraid to say how excited you are to know so many other men will look at her, wanting her.

Now is the time to be more explicit in discussing things that may have felt awkward talking about in the initial stages of your cuckold journey. Don't be afraid to tell her you adore it when she gets frustrated that you're soft or too small to please her. Tell her you appreciate it when she says things like you're a wimp.

Vocalize your desire to see her more demanding, selfish, or even better, bitchy. It will feel scary being so open and honest in areas that may still feel "off" to what is considered normal. But let's face it, cuckolding at no level is "normal". It's way beyond normal. By the time you get to this point, if you've followed all the other steps first, it will not be as uncomfortable a conversation as if you've fast-tracked to just reading this before doing everything else first.

What you're trying to accomplish in this step is letting her know the direction you are both heading is working... at least for you. See if her feedback suggests she is uncomfortable taking things further or wants to stay where you are in the dynamic for a while longer. NEVER PUSH. Until she is ready to move on to the next step, just enjoy the changes that have already taken place and know she is a lot closer to becoming your Goddess than she was at the start.

If you both agree that things seem to be good, ask her if she's given any more thought about taking things outside of the relationship in real terms. This is a key opportunity to get her attention, by the way. If you suspect the only thing stopping her from saying "yes" is her fear you might get upset, have the conversation ONLY when you are in a compromised position.

"Compromised position?"

Yup. Either when you are both in bed (nude) or when you are wearing something that allows easy access of her hand.

As she is disclosing to you she likes the idea, or that she's enjoyed being selfish or finds being a bitch natural - take her hand and place it on your pathetic and useless piece of equipment. If you're a cuckold, I don't think I need to say anything else here.

Seeing and/or feeling how "happy" and excited you are will be the catalyst to push her over the edge. If you both have the internal green light, it is now time to take things up and out to the real world. You are now ready to start the real journey of cuckolding.

STEP 11 - FLIRT TILL IT HURTS

---

o you're now a cuckold couple (that hasn't cuckolded yet) out in the real world. What do you do now? Find a bull and say "Here look, honey. Here's a guy you can fuck."? Do that and you have wasted all your efforts to evolve into a healthy cuckold relationship that is supportive, loving, and LASTING.

Things still need to move at a snail's pace. This is where things get real. For both of you. Up till now, it has all been in your head. As soon as you add another human being to the mix, it becomes a reality that can never be undone. Both of you need to be very sensitive to this concept and move at a mutually comfortable pace.

Just as in the beginning stages of introducing your Goddess to a disparity in the home took baby steps, the same is applicable here. Baby steps start with one small first step. What is that first step you ask? The innocent but very real process of outward, overt, and intentional flirting. Nothing big. Just flirting. Simple right?

For me, this was harder than going down on a guy. By the time I did that, I knew davie would be in heaven. But flirting is the 'outside world' first step that is a lot more uncomfortable and nerve-wracking.

It does not have to be elaborate or done in any special or specific way. It just needs to be done. She needs to do it. And you need to be right there, beside her, as it's happening.

Why?

THIS IS THE FIRST OUTWARD ACT you will have as a cuckold couple. Your Goddess will have to overcome the nervousness she'll feel about your reaction. She'll have to overcome any residual feelings of guilt that she may not realize are still living deep in her old-fashioned values. On the other hand, you'll have to deal with the mild forms of anger, jealousy, angst (and of course, excitement). And with you being there, you'll face dealing with the embarrassment you'll feel in front of another man now flirting with "your woman".

I know it seems so small and innocent, but once you're there, at the moment - a sudden wave of thoughts, reactions, and emotions will come out of nowhere that neither of you would have expected. Play it out. Feel everything. No actual lines have been crossed. This is an excellent test to see if you want to move forward or not. In the context of this book, it becomes your first chance to show how much you want, approve, and arguably need cuckolding to form the predominant dynamic within your relationship together.

Try to appreciate how powerful these first "innocent"

flirting actions have on your partner's acceptance and embracement of the lifestyle. If she sees you have no problems, with a gigantic smile on your face and a massively heightened attentiveness to her needs? She'll feel on top of the world. Like she can do no wrong. This is a big push for her. It opens the door wide. Now you both just need to walk around inside.

You should note that having a debriefing after this step is essential to both of you. That is once you're back in the privacy and safety of your own home. You need to talk about how you both felt. What you didn't like? What did she feel uncomfortable with? How did it make you feel? You want to lay everything on the table. As I assume you can guess, there isn't much left in the way of testing for each of you.

If she feels good, use this event to dig into how much more alive and happy you felt watching her talk and flirt with another man. Reassure her it was not just ok with you, it was friggen amazing.

The extent of flirting, and for how long - depends on each couple. I would encourage you both to take this kind of innocent fun as far as you can. She may only feel confident to smile and eye fuck a man across the room at first. Not much, but it's a start. This kind of thing not only helps to break the ice, but it circumvents some emotionally charged realities you both need to face head-on.

Suggest going to a nite-club together. Have her go to the bar to get your drinks and then start up a flirty conversation with Mr. Big. Make sure you're in the middle of the exchange once they talk. You want to let your Goddess see you're aware and okay with her actions. It will also give you a chance to stand there, all prissy with your umbrella drink, listening to them talk while you just take it like a little girl. Humiliating? Uncomfortable? Goes against the normal reaction that you feel yourself fighting? Yes, yes, and yes.

Is there a big bulge in your pants? Is your heart racing with excitement? Are you looking at your partner, thinking how wonderful she is to do this to you? LET HER KNOW. As your comfort level goes up, let her know as it's happening IN FRONT OF Mr. Big. I've always found it a little sexy when davie helps put my real man at ease.

STEP 12 - BABY STEPS OUTSIDE

tep 12. I thought it would fit to make this a "12-step". (no disrespect to any AA readers, just a little twisted humor from my end)

This is where the point of no return is crossed. If you are here, you're looking for ways to help ease the final transition into cuckolding and helping your Goddess feel like the path is not only the right direction, it's the only direction for you both to be happy and fulfilled as a couple.

As with every other step, the transition to this must be mutual and non-threatening. Don't plan an elaborate meet-up at a hotel with some random bull your Cuckoldress met on some online chat or dating website. That kind of scenario makes for way too much pressure and stress for anyone to have a good time. As she gains experience and confidence, this is a probable option (particularly with bulls already established - speaking from my experience) but not at the early stages.

Look for ways to help your partner feel relaxed, safe, and supported by you. I've mentioned this before but it's worth mentioning again - swinger clubs. Yes, they cater to couples looking to hook-up with other couples. But there is no rule everyone has to play. They are packed with open-minded, non-judgemental, and sexually adventurous peeps. Dress codes are very provocative and the intended point of "cumming" is, well... you get it. No one is there to meet Mr. or Miss Right. Sexual pleasure is king.

Let your Cuckoldress move at her own speed. Tell her you would love to see her make out with this guy or that. If she says she thinks the dude in the corner is hot, make her a bet. Bet her a drink that she can't get her hands down his pants to make him hard. Yes, this is a kind of childish behavior, but you are both going to be nervous. Especially your partner. Betting her to put her hand on another man's cock, or to have a kissing make-out session... it's not sex, but it is way past anything she would have dreamed of doing when you first started talking about her being "the boss" in the household.

You don't need me to give you a play-by-play on fore-play. Just know that your need to see her reach complete ecstasy is a lot closer than you think at this point. The touching, kissing, rubbing - they are all windows behind the door you opened earlier. All that's waiting is for her to feel safe in the environment, safe with whomever she is now playing with, and safe in her relationship with you.

Now more than ever, you need to encourage her. Don't be afraid to be strong in your words. Saying "I would love to see you suck his cock or get your brains fucked silly by him"... She needs to hear that. She's already thinking it herself, BELIEVE ME.

You are the last roadblock before things go under the sheets.

Of almost equal importance is aftercare. How you respond once they do the deed can have a massive positive or destructive effect on things going deeper or evaporating into thin air. I remember feeling sooooooo guilty for the first time. I looked for davie, feeling mortified with myself and praying he would forgive me for getting lost in the moment.

Had he been anything less than happy, excited, and encouraging would have torn me apart. I needed to know he was not upset or didn't think less of me. His first words besides "You're amazing. I'm so lucky to have you," were "I'd love if you could do that again. Actually, I'd love if we could kind of make this our lifestyle."

It sold me. I think we fucked till sunrise once we got home. It was amazing. And yes, his reaction very much helped increase my desire to pursue this as a relationship dynamic. His words also helped me accept I am who I am... a cuckoldress. I stopped fighting myself and gave in to my desires. Every time was easier, more enjoyable, and more seductive to want to go further. I wanted to be the boss. I wanted to control him. I wanted to fuck who and when I pleased. And the groundwork laid out in this book also made me learn to accept davie and to understand I also wanted to humiliate him. He loved it, which made me love him even more (if that's even possible).

The caveat?

Cuckold angst. I don't get it myself. But davie has spent many hours trying to help me understand it. Be careful of the aftercare and your responses and reactions to your cuckoldress. This will be the real beginning of your cuck relationship. Everything before will help bring your spouse to the emotional and physical understanding that it's okay and that it's something you want. But suddenly, out of nowhere, you're going to have a bunch of negative emotions. Some may throw you in a pit of depression or anger. If you let your cuckoldress see even a hint of this, you're done.

If you want greater clarity on what it is or how to deal with it, check out my DNA - Husband Edition book. Going into the mechanics here is outside the scope of this book. Suffice to say, you are 100% guaranteed going to experience this. You also have no way to predict when or in what ways it will affect you. If you want your relationship to form a long-term cuckold dynamic (or I would argue, you don't want it... You need it) with the woman you have just taken this 12 step journey with; you need to squash it like a bug.

Do not UNDER ANY CIRCUMSTANCES let her see this side of you in the initial stages of her becoming a cuckoldress. If you do, you must acknowledge you are not a cuckold, for it will surely put the chances of the dynamic into outer space.

As you grow together as a cuckold couple... I just love the sound of that. Davie and I are a cuckold couple. Sexy, right? As you grow together, over time, then you can express your angst so she understands when you seem a bit "off" from time to time. I've been told that the angst transitions into a good thing. You crave it. What do I know? I just crave the cock.

FINAL THOUGHTS

ow does one summarize a topic that is so complex and varied from couple to couple? Patience, understanding, compliance, and communication.

You need all four.

But there is a secret missing ingredient. Love.

If you approach cuckolding from a place of love, you can not go wrong. And this love starts at the beginning of the journey. If your wife is just not interested in cuckolding at any level, could you push, manipulate and get your way, anyway? Possibly. But this is not a man who loves his wife if he would do such a thing.

I fear some readers may have this book, looking for ways to trick or manipulate their spouse into cuckolding because it gets them off. Not cool! Your spouse is an actual human being with genuine emotions and a heart. This is a journey you must take together.

I have seen a plethora of books, movies, and other media that offer the illusion that there is some magical way to "convert/convince/seduce" your wife into a cuckoldress. This is not for everyone. Many women don't have a high enough sex drive to warrant this lifestyle or don't have the moral fortitude to get over the social stigma.

This book is for any couple that would not fall into the above. It's for the cuck hubby whose wife has perhaps foo foo'd the idea a bit? Maybe she is scared cause it's so out there... but she is curious? Maybe for the man that instinctively knows his wife wants this life but is too ashamed or afraid to admit it to him, even after he's disclosed his desires to be cuckolded? This is not a manual of deception or manipulation.

If, at the end of your journey along these steps, your wife says "stop" or decides she has given further consideration and is not interested in pursuing it, please respect her wishes. Failure to do so is a failure to love. If her lack of desire or willingness causes problems for you in the bedroom, seek outside professional help. There are always solutions. Most are in fact just outside your own sphere of knowledge or understanding.

For your wife to transition into a cuckoldress, you both will undergo many levels of change - with yourselves and with each other. The framework laid out here is unlike any of the other information you may come across in this area. No hardcore, graphic tips to do this or that are offered. It's a gentle, soft, and slow transition. Why? Because I know this lifestyle has the potential to be amazing. BUT, it has the same potential to end your marriage in a matter of months. Davie and I have seen it happen, and it breaks our hearts when it happens.

IF YOUR WIFE IS ON THE FENCE, the information offered above will probably push her over the edge. Under any other circumstances, you don't need this book - you're already there... or it will never happen (because she is not interested, and you have ethics).

For me, the biggest struggles surrounded guilt and fear that I would hurt little davie's heart. For some of my cuckoldress friends, it was suffering from low self-esteem - feeling that they didn't deserve to be treated like a Goddess. And still, for others, it was rationalizing how increasing disparity could be a positive and enjoyable experience for them and their cuckold husbands.

The steps I've offered, deal with each of the above potential objections in a progressive and logical fashion. We need step 1 for step 2. Step 2 builds a foundation to move to step 3... and so on. You don't need to follow the steps sequentially, but from my experience, it is the natural flow of progression as you grow into a cuckold couple. As with all relationships, everyone is different and what works for one may be less effective or require less or more time than another. The point is, you need to move slow and understand it is not an end-game process. The magic of cuckolding is the journey you both take AS A COUPLE. To see your wife evolve into a sexual goddess that becomes all-powerful over you and your life **BECAUSE SHE WANTS TO**... **NOT because you made her.**

I have a couple of loose end admin things. If you have found this book to be helpful, please take a minute and give it a rating from whatever book retailer you purchased it. Even better, leave a comment. It helps others find the content that helps our community grow.

One last thing. As with my DNA series, I am now

working on the female companion book to this - to help women learn what buttons to push to help their man transition into a soft, gentle, and obedient cuckold. If your wife wants to push you (and you want to be pushed into the cuck life), but she doesn't know how - this is the book for her.

H ugs and kisses,

A and d

ALSO BY ALLORA SINCLAIR

ABOUT THE AUTHOR

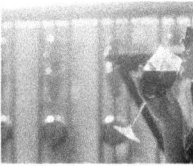

ABOUT THE AUTHOR

Allora Sinclair is a happily married 40 year old mom. She and her loving cuckold husband Dave (davie) have been in a cuckold marriage for over seven years and she has now decided to start documenting their journey. If Allora is not found at her computer or out shopping for a new pair of shoes, she is usually found in the caring arms of davie or embraced in ecstasy with one of her favorite bulls. She has done a series of non-fiction books to help couples navigate their way through the heavily distorted life of being a cuckold couple. She has also worked on a series of fiction books that are loosely based on some of their real-life adventures. If you found this book to be of value, please be sure to rate it or leave a comment with the book retailer you got it from.

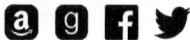

www.ingramcontent.com/pod-product-compliance
Lightning Source LLC
Chambersburg PA
CBHW070817280326
41934CB00012B/3212